How

to lose

weight

without medication

Ben Williams

DEDICATION

To you, you and you fighting against obesity

Preface

This book will be discussing extensively on how to lose weight safely without medication and the important of nutrient to the body system. This book is projected to reveal the damage done to your body system by trying to cut excess weight with the use of hard drugs.

CONTENTS

humans and body weight

Body weight varies throughout the day, this is due to variation in water contents of the body at the different times of the day. It can also be a result of human activities such as drinking, urinating, and sweating.

Drinking can affect the weight of human by adding more weight to the ideal body weight of human while urinating affect the weight of human by reducing the ideal weight. You will agree with me that during exercises human system undergoes the process of dehydration, this allows the system to give out water through sweat thereby the weight of that individual is reduced if you are watchful enough you notice a drastic change in weight because the system has lost some amount of water. If actually, you want to reduce your weight for some individual purposes, it's advisable you adopt a method called weighting cutting so as to maintain ideal fat for a healthy living. Weight cutting is the practice of fast weight loss in a particular period of time. There two methods by which this process can be practiced,

- Losing weight in form of fat and muscle in a specific period

- This involves losing weight in form of water in a given period of time.

Achieving and maintain the ideal body weight takes some serious commitment but reaching a healthy weight can be beneficial for your overall weight, excess weight increases the chances for developing some health problem such as diabetes, high blood pressure, and cancer. in the year 2014 research shows that 34.9% America adult is obese if we want our body system to be free from being overweight there are things we need to know or do in all ramification of our daily life. The ways in which we feed, the way in which we excise our body and the type of food we eat and the food content must be looked into for the benefit of the healthier living.

Find out the number of calories you need in your body system. to consume a right amount of calories you should determine the basal metabolic rate that will enable you to know the right amount of calories that your body system needs to function while putting to rest. You can also track the number of calories in your body system, you must learn how to eat to lose weight and also ensure you are not eating a higher amount of calories or a lesser amount of calories require by the body system. If eventually, you are eating more calories you can either add walkout to your day or reduce the number of calories you take into your system.

Effects of overweight on the human body

In the year2003 statistics shown that about one billion adults is considered to be obese, also in the year 2013 statistics show that there is a double increase in the number of obese as a result of careless method of our diet. This is another broad day enemy that is sending many people to an early grave, render them useless or making them look unattractive.

Excess weight is the un ideal weight that makes an individual look unhealthy, unattractive, ill relevant and unhappy especially among the female. one of the way that can make you look attractive and healthy is to maintain an ideal weight. If you must do this you need a diligent approach to achieve a better result.

Losing weight is not as easy or as quick as you may think, there are things you must do or there are sacrifices you must pay if you must achieve a good result such as avoiding some kind of foods for a healthier and attractive look. You must avoid some food that gives unnecessary fat like sugary cereal, its taste nice, yes I know it also looks attractive, yes I know but let me tell you they do more harm than good in the body system try as much as possible to put them out of your reach. Cereal is made from ultra-refined grain but cereal is high in calories and tends to be high in sugary, many cereals have as much sugar as a glazed donut.granted, calories wise, much high fiber cereals like fiber one is fairly low in energy, however, the more popular cereal that people that people actually eat are not low calories food. Cereal also activates brain chemical that makes you feel sedated. in often times we had misconception that cereal energizes your body system which is not always true, cereal stimulate an inhibitory system of transmitter in the brain, making the body system feel sedated and sleepy.incontrast food that is high in amino acids, such as quality protein stimulate the brain cells to keep you alert and vigilant. Cereal is so dangerous to body system because they have low-quality protein since it is made predominately from refined grains which are carbohydrate. However, there are many other foods that we can consume without exposing us to health threat such as protein in natural form.

Writing out a plan on how to excesses during the week and a meal plan, this helps greatly by committing yourself to achieve a good result. Eating healthy and exercise can seem like a pretty simple and straightforward goal, however, there are many different components to a healthy diet and fitness program. You need to choose a particular day of the week for walking out and also choose what food to eat, when to eat the food and how to prepare them. Starting with a specific goal and detail plan can help you implement the change you need you to need to help you eat healthier. Use food recall method to achieve this goal by planning what you eat and drink on a particular day in all your meals.

Always take your breakfast on regular basis, drink less soda and eat more vegetables. Eat enough vegetables and fruits because fruits and vegetables are of low calories and high in fibers, vitamins and minerals. it's also important you choose fruits and vegetable that are most nutrients dense. Physical activities are also of a great advantage to achieve a good result because through these process a certain amount of water and nutrient goes out of the body system through sweat. Such as gyms, swimming, dancing, hiking, walking etc.

Don't deprive yourself of any meal especially breakfast because breakfast is responsible for putting our metabolism in action for the day. The longer breakfast is delayed the longer it takes for metabolism to take place in order to burn fat in the body system, take light food as breakfast so as to start metabolism without overloading it with calories. Take more water with the low amount of calories such as sad because this can prevent several hundred of calories from going into the body system.

chew slowly whenever you are eating food and make sure all your food are finely mused not only does this in the digestive system but it makes you full easily, the reason for this is that if the food is chewed stay chunky through digestion and build up in the stomach area.

Eat slowly because it takes the brain up to 20 minutes to send a message to the system that you ate, so if slowly you are eating by the time you finished the message is sent and you will not eat an unnecessary extra serving.

Overweight and diabetes

Overweight and obesity are all risk factors for developing type 2 diabetes. Most times, individuals are not aware of the health risk of overweight until they are diagnosed with pre-diabetes or type 2 diabetes. Diabetes is a chronic, potentially debilitating that need medical attention and monitoring of an individual's blood sugar level and treatment. In type 2 diabetes, the body does not produce or use insulin, a hormone produced by the pancreas that help in the circulation of sugar into cells. The body then becomes resistant to insulin. This resistance cause's high blood sugar levels. High amount of sugar in the blood causes many health-related challenges. The cells find it difficult to get enough of the sugar they need,

And when the amount of sugar in the blood become too high, it damage the nerves and blood vessels, usually in the heart, feet, hands, kidneys and eyes. another problem of high percentage of sugar and insulin resistance include: Increased risk of heart disease and stroke Neuropathy (nerve damage, especially in extremities) Nephropathy (renal impairment, kidney failure) Retinopathy (vision problems, blindness) cardiovascular disease (heart disease and increased risk of stroke) erectile dysfunction in men and reduce sexual desire ingot men and women. between meals, the body may depend on stored glucose in the liver glycogen for energy. Glycogen is made up of several thousand glucose molecules held together with water molecules. If the fast is very long, however, the body will instead use amino acids or fatty acids to help with its metabolic processes. After taking a meal, the processes of chewing and chemical digestion glucose is produced(sugar), that is always available as fuel for our organs especially muscle and brain tissue. In a normal circumstances , the glucose produced from these digestive processes go into our cells to help with other metabolic processes. Insulin acts a key that open the door to let glucose in to feed our cells. When insulin is present, it also put off the process of using glycogen from the liver to ensure that the glucose level does not go beyond after a meal. In fact, insulin reduces blood glucose by collecting any excess glucose that is available in the blood stream so that it can be stored as glycogen for future use. However, if the require amount of insulin is not available, as is the case in diabetes, then this glucose is unable to go into the cells. Instead, the glucose stays in the blood stream in a higher portion of usual concentration. This condition is known as elevated blood glucose or hyperglycemia.

Exercise can also be a useful tool to reduce blood glucose levels. When we use our muscles, they need more fuel to stay alive. In patients without diabetes, glucose is taken into the body system from the blood stream while a simultaneous rise in the liver's glucose production keep the muscles supplied with fuel. However, when type 2 diabetes is available in a particular body, the liver may not match the muscle's need for glucose, which can result in a lowering of the glucose level with moderate exercise. Thus, exercise is widely recommended to treat patients with high sugar level.

Excess weight can greatly affect your health in various ways, with type 2 diabetes being one of the most serious. There are various forms of measurement used to check someone's excess weight; however, the most commonly -used method is knowing your body mass index through calculation. There are five weight status categories that any living person may fit into:

Underweight

Normal weight

Overweight

Obesity

Severe obesity

When an individual predisposed to diabetes has excess Weight, the body cells become less active to the insulin that is released from the pancreas. There are some proves that fat cells are more resistant to insulin than muscle cells. Individuals affected by type 2 diabetes, who exercise, appear to reduce the severity of insulin-resistance because the exercising muscles use the extra sugar found in the blood; as a result of this , the body does not secrete insulin and the sugar is no longer diverted to excess fat cells. It's not just how much an individual I weighs, but also where they carry the weight that puts them at greater risk for health problems. Individuals carrying more weight around their waist are more likely to suffer from obesity-related conditions than someone who carries more weight in their hips and thighs. Individual that are affected by excess weight, mostly obesity and severe obesity, are more likely to develop type 2 diabetes as a related condition of their excess weight. Obesity and severe obesity greatly increase your risk of developing heart disease, type 2 diabetes, certain types of cancer, sleep apnea, osteoarthritis and much more. To know your body mass index and determine your weight status category. You Are at risk for type 2 diabetes? What you eat on a daily basis and how active you are affects your risk of developing type 2 diabetes. Being overweight (body mass index of 25-29.9 or affected by obesity body mass index of 30-39.9 or severe obesity, body mass index of 40 or greater, greatly increases your risk of developing type 2 diabetes. The higher excess weight present in your body system, the more resistant your muscle and tissue cells become to your own insulin hormone. Over 90 percent of people with type 2 diabetes are overweight or affected by a degree of obesity. In addition to excess weight, there are other various factors that increase your risk of developing type 2 diabetes, such as:

Sedentary Lifestyle, lack of exercise and having excess weight overweight go hand-in- hand with a diagnosis of type 2 diabetes. Muscle cells have more insulin receptors than fat cells, so an individual can reduce insulin resistance by exercising. Being more active also reduces blood sugar levels by making insulin to be more effective.

Unhealthy eating is a contributor to obesity. High amount of fat in your diet, not enough fiber and too many simple carbohydrates all contribute to the development of type 2 diabetes. Family History and Genetics, It appears that people who have family members with type 2 diabetes are at a higher risk for developing it themselves. As we age, the risk of type 2 diabetes becomes higher . Even if an elderly person is not big in size, they still may be predisposed to developing diabetes. The pancreas ages right along with us and doesn't pump insulin as efficiently as it did when we were younger. As our cells age, they become more resistant to insulin as well. High Blood Pressure and High Cholesterol are the main causes of Diseases and health challenges, including type 2 diabetes. Not only do they destroy heart vessels, but they are two key components in metabolic syndrome, a cluster of sign including obesity, a high fat diet and lack of exercise. Having metabolic syndrome increases the risk of heart disease, stroke and type 2 diabetes.

Women affected by obesity are more insulin resistant when compared to women of an ideal weight. When pregnant, gestational diabetes generally last for the period of pregnancy and approximately 5 to 10 percent of women with gestational diabetes will continually affected by diabetes even after delivery. How do you detect type 2 diabetes? There are different type of blood tests that may show whether you have type 2 diabetes or not. Let's take a look at each test and see what different results could mean for you and your health. Fasting Blood Sugar Chart

Sugar Level Indicates

Under 100 mg/dL = Normal

100 to 125 mg/dL = Prediabetes

126 mg/dL and above = Diabetes

Fasting Blood Sugar Level Chart

Blood Sugar level HGbA1c Indicates

Under 100 mg/dL Normal

100 to 125 mg/dL Pre-diabetes

126 mg/dL or higher on 2 separate tests Diabetes

Fasting Blood Sugar Test, The amount of sugar present in your blood is naturally not stable but stays within a normal range. The preferred way to check your blood sugar level is after fasting overnight for at least eight hours. A fasting blood sugar level less than 100 milligrams of sugar per deciliter of blood is considered normal. If your blood sugar level measures from 100 to 125, you have impaired fasting glucose, and this may be a sign that you have pre-diabetes. If your blood sugar level is more than 200 mg/dL , with signs of diabetes.

EXERCISE AND ITS POSITIVE VIBES

Research has shown the benefit of a good exercise, good exercise doesn't only help in managing your weight it also minimixe your risk of developing heart diseases. it increase your good living and also activate our good mood. Irrespective of your age exercise play a vital role in maintaining an ideal weight and also makes you look more active. in 2012 research has shown that over 30% of children aged two to fifteen are now classed as either overweight or obese. However, it's very important you get involves in active physical activities. Good execs affect your life positively in the following ways

It stimulates the development of the muscles, bones, joints as well as heart and lungs.

It helps you maintain a healthy weight

It gives you an opportunity to interact with other people which help in the development of your brain.

It helps in managing symptoms of anxiety and depression.

There are many different exercise options to be involved in. going for gym or heading out to run is not the only exercise you can do, it may be as simple as walking to and from the shop instead of getting a drop/taxi, dancing, swimming cycling skipping etc. If you have not been doing exercise or if you have stop for a while now it's going to be of a great benefit for you to get back to the field and get started.

It is very necessary for you keep your heart healthy, Exercise is one of best things you can use to keep your heart healthy and reduce your risk of developing stroke and coronary heart diseases. In the UK almost every year over 4100 people dies from stroke and around 74,000 from coronary heart diseases. Regular exercise help to reduce high blood pressure which is very common among the adult in our society today, which can influence stroke or heart failure. exercise also help in improving the balance of your cholesterol.

It's estimated that around 3.2 million people in the UK have diabetes; regular physical activities help to reduce the rate at which you have it. Obesity is a major factor for diabetes. Exercise regularly help you to maintain a healthy weight and therefore reduce your risk of becoming overweight or obese which can lead to type 2 diabetes. Physical activities burn up calories and help to create a healthy energy balance. as such it is good you always go for a brisk walk in nearby woodlands or a park, only you reap the physical benefits but being outside surrounded by nature and beautiful scenery can do your wellbeing and health wonders.

DIETING AND WEIGHT LOSS

It's very annoying to feel like you are overweighing not t o talk of the health challenges involved. it makes you fee l sluggish and less confidence of yourself. one of the best way to look smart and healthier is to review what you co nsume and also control the portion size.

Diet is always most effective when combined with other healthy lifestyle choice and good aptitude. If we must m aintain a good diet there are some compulsory attitude t hat we must adopt in order to have a good result. You m ust check the way at which you eat presently because w e can't continue to be doing some certain things in the s ame way and expect a different result so as a result of th is you must check your current eating habit. at this point it's advisable you have your own food roster, adopt the method of using food journal in the kitchen which will cl early state the type of food you are to eat on daily basis and it must not be compromised. Identify what triggers your overfeeding habit such as stress, fatigue loneliness, excessive hunger, etc. for the fact that you have been ab le to identify this problem, you are moving to the directi on where you will experience a turnaround in your diet. When we feel under the gun or anxious, we often turn t o food for comfort which may lead us to overfeed oursel

ves, if this is what triggers your overfeeding you then ne
ed to include stress management techniques. Loneliness
can also make you overfeed yourself if you are the type t
hat falls back to food or make food your friend wheneve
r you are bored it's advisable at this point you think of a
nother hubby to supplement food to enable you to over
come this problem.

MEASURING YOUR BODY FAT

Body fat percentage is the amount of fat present in the b ody of an individual in percentage. it comprises of the es sential fat and storage fat. They can be found in the nerv es, bone marrow, and body organs. Storage body fat acc umulates as a result of excess energy or calories that are being consumed You can safely reduce this fat to either l ose weight or lower your body fat percentage.

U.S Navy has come up with a method of calculating your body percentage which involves mathematics and meas urement in order to give your insight in your weight as a function of your health, in doing this you need just some few instruments such as measuring tape, calculator mea suring scale etc.

The first step you need to do is to measure your height with the use of measuring tape. You have to stand uprig ht and take off your shoe for an accurate result after whi ch you measure your waist with the same accuracy proc ess then you measure the neck, for accuracy sake also ke ep your head straight and look forward and make sure y our shoulders are down and relax and also measure your hips (female only) after you might have gotten all these values then, for male %body fat = 86.010*log10 (waist-n eck)-70.041*log10 (height) +36.76.

Female %body fat = 163.205*log10 (waist +hip-neck)-97.684*log10 (height)-97.387.

HUMAN WEIGHT AND BLOOD PRESSURE

High Blood pressure is one of the most common health c hallenges in our society today, in the year 2016 statistics have shown that about 75 million American adults (32%) have high blood pressure that is one in every three yout h. This health challenge is needed to be treated with me dication unless it can be controlled by lifestyle changes.

However, you must learn to do away with excessive tabl e salt (NaCl) you only need small quantity of table salt in your food. sodium is responsible for the regulation of ele ctrical processes in the nerves and muscle which excess of it can make you retain excess fluid that will make your blood have more volume, this will cause your heart to p ump harder to move that excess fluid around the body. This usually results in high blood pressure. Research has shown that people eat about 3,500 mg of sodium per da y. The dash diet which is short for a dietary approach to stop hypertension recommends no more than 2,300mg of sodium per day.

Dairy is the major source of calcium and vitamin, howev er, it's important to choose carefully the kind of dairy pr oducts you consume because of its high content of salt a nd fat. Whenever you take cheese and yogurt go for the low fat and low salt respectively. You also need to reduc e the quantity of sugar consumption. Sugar only add calories to your diet and make you feel satisfied without add nutrient to your body. Alcohol does more harm than good to your body system because of its calories and sugar content, it's going to be of a great benefit to you if the level of your alcoholic intake is reduced. Much intake of any alcoholic substance prone you to obesity. You can lower your blood pressure by quitting drinking or drinking only in moderation.

CALCULATE YOUR BLOOD VOLUME.

It's very necessary to calculate your blood volume so as t
o know the volume of anesthesia you may need in case
of any surgery or to make sure that you are not donating
more than its safe for you during blood donation. There
are many ways of calculating blood volume and there m
ay be slightly different but there should be no much diff
erence in the result.

Remember I said there are various ways that you can us
e to calculate your blood volume. For the sake of my rea
ders were going to be using one of the simplest methods
where we will be using Nadler equation, in this method,
blood volume is going to be calculated in millimeters. Be
fore this calculation can be done you need to know your
height value (inches) and your weight(pounds) then mult
iply 0.006012 by the value of your height and multiply 1
4.6 by the value of your weight add both of them togeth
er and also add 604 to your final answer.

www.ingramcontent.com/pod-product-compliance
Lightning Source LLC
Chambersburg PA
CBHW051428250726

48655CB00003B/1296